FAST FACTS

WP 166

Gynaecological Oncology

‖‖‖‖‖‖‖‖‖‖‖‖‖‖‖‖‖
00657349

Indispensable

Guides to

Clinical

Practice

J Richard Smith

Consultant in Gynaecology, Honorary Senior
Lecturer in Obstetrics and Gynaecology,
Imperial College School of Medicine at
Chelsea and Westminster Hospital,
London, UK, and Visiting Professor,
New York Medical Center, New York, USA

Bruce A Barron

Professor of Clinical Gynecology, Columbia
University College of Physicians and Surgeons,
and Attending Physician, The Presbyterian
Hospital in the City of New York,
New York, USA

Andrew D Lawson (CHAPTER 6)

Consultant in Pain Management,
Chelsea and Westminster Hospital,
London, UK

THE ROYAL OLDHAM HOSPITAL
MEDICAL LIBRARY

HEALTH PRESS

Oxford

Fast Facts – Gynaecological Oncology
First published 1998

© 1998 Health Press Limited
Elizabeth House, Queen Street, Abingdon
Oxford, UK, OX14 3JR
Tel: +44 (0)1235 523233
Fax: +44 (0)1235 523238

Fast Facts is a trademark of Health Press Limited.

All rights reserved. No part of this publication may be reproduced,
stored in a retrieval system, or transmitted in any form or by any
means, electronic, mechanical, photocopying, recording or
otherwise, without the express permission of the publisher.

The Right of J Richard Smith and Bruce A Barron to be identified
as the Authors of this Work has been asserted in accordance with
the Copyright, Designs & Patents Act 1988 Sections 77 and 78.

The publisher, the authors, and Wyeth Laboratories have made
every effort to ensure the accuracy of this book, but cannot accept
responsibility for any errors or omissions. A CIP catalogue record
for this title is available from the British Library.

ISBN 1-899541-36-5

Library of Congress
Cataloging-in-Publication Data

Smith, JR, (J Richard)
Fast Facts – Gynaecological Oncology/
J Richard Smith, Bruce A Barron

Illustrated by MeDee Art, London UK
Printed by Fine Print, Oxford, UK

Abbreviations

Beta-HCG: beta-human chorionic gonadotrophin

Ca 125: a tumour marker

CIN: cervical intraepithelial neoplasia

ECS: endocervical swab

EUA: examination under anaesthesia

GTN: gestational trophoblastic neoplasia

HPV: human papillomavirus

HSV: herpes simplex virus

HVS: high vaginal swab

IMB: intermenstrual bleeding

LLETZ: large loop excision of the transformation zone

LMP: last menstrual period

PCB: postcoital bleeding

STD: sexually transmitted disease

VAIN: vaginal intraepithelial neoplasia

VE: vaginal examination

VIN: vulval intraepithelial neoplasia

Introduction

Gynaecological oncology is a well-established subspecialty of gynaecology. Management of gynaecological malignancy is shared between the gynaecologist, radiotherapist, medical oncologist, family physician and, occasionally, the palliative care specialist. Women have become increasingly aware of their risk of genital tract malignancy, particularly as a result of the cervical screening programme, the increasing publicity given to attempts to develop screening tests for ovarian cancer, and the increased risk of endometrial cancer among women receiving either hormone replacement therapy, or tamoxifen for breast cancer.

The incidence of cervical cancer is declining in industrialized countries, almost certainly due to the implementation of cervical smear programmes. It remains true, however, that those women most in need of screening are those least likely to be included in programmes, and there is still much room for improvement.

At present, 21 000 new cases of ovarian cancer are diagnosed each year in the USA, and approximately 13 000 deaths occur annually. This disease accounts for 4% of all tumours in women.

Gynaecological tumours that have a low incidence are seen infrequently by the non-subspecialist, but nevertheless require prompt recognition and management to minimize their potentially devastating effects.

Fast Facts – Gynaecological Oncology aims to update the family physician and non-specialist who see these tumours infrequently, on current management and prognosis. It should also provide a useful starting point for junior doctors on a gynaecological oncology rotation.

CHAPTER 1

Cervical cancer

Epidemiology

The incidence of cervical cancer in the general population is uncertain, but is probably 8–10 women/100 000/year. The incidence varies with geographic area. Cervical cancer is more common in metropolitan areas than in rural areas, and the incidence is higher in populations with lower socio-economic status.

Epidemiologically, smoking has been shown to be implicated in this disease and laboratory evidence suggests this may be mediated via its effects on Langerhans' cells, the local immune cells in the cervix. In addition, generalized immunosuppression, either iatrogenically stimulated (e.g. post-renal transplantation) or as a result of HIV infection, has been shown to predispose to cervical intraepithelial neoplasia (CIN) – the precancerous state.

Aetiology

Cervical squamous carcinoma and its precursor, CIN, have multifactorial aetiology. Their development is related to sexual activity. Human papillomaviruses (HPV), particularly types 16, 18, 31, 33, 51 and 54, have been implicated in the development of cervical cancer. In the past, herpes simplex virus (HSV) was thought to be an aetiological factor, but this has now been questioned. An association has been demonstrated between CIN and the woman's age, age at first sexual intercourse, and the total number of sexual partners a woman has had. There may be a 'male factor' involved; some men have been shown to have had a number of partners who developed CIN, and semen appears to have a number of local immunosuppressive qualities.

The mechanism for development of CIN is probably:

- infection with HPV
- integration of HPV into the host cell genome
- transformation of the cell by HPV, probably with the assistance of co-factors (e.g. generalized or local immunosuppression).

CIN has been shown to be the precursor of invasive cervical neoplasia.

CIN 1 progresses to cervical cancer in about 1% of cases, and review of the literature reveals an overall range of progression varying from 1.4% to 60%. More than 15% of women with CIN 3 will develop invasive cervical cancer in 10 years, and 20–30% will develop it in 20 years. There is much variation in approach to the management of CIN 1 and borderline smears in both the UK and USA. The Papanicolaou system of CIN classification into borderline, 1, 2 and 3 has certain disadvantages. Some authors have suggested that the Bethesda system, namely low grade (CIN 1 and 2) and high grade (CIN 2 and 3), would be more reproducible.

The area of the cervix with premalignant potential is the transformation zone, and is formed after puberty. Before puberty, the squamocolumnar junction is found inside the endocervical canal (Figure 1.1a); at puberty, cervical eversion occurs under the influence of oestrogens, resulting in cervical ectopy (Figure 1.1b). The vagina is then colonized by lactobacilli and the acidity increases. This encourages squamous cell metaplasia, covering the area of cervical ectopy (columnar epithelium) with squamous epithelium (Figure 1.1c). Thus, there are two squamocolumnar junctions: the original one and the new one (Figure 1.1d). The area between these is the transformation zone, and it is this area that has premalignant potential. It is also this area that must be investigated using cervical cytology. After the menopause, the new squamocolumnar junction ascends into the cervical canal (Figure 1.1e).

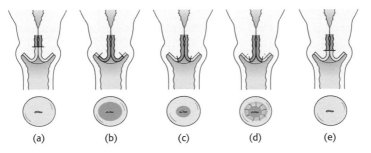

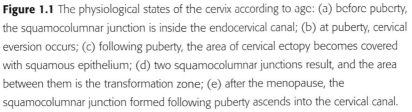

Figure 1.1 The physiological states of the cervix according to age: (a) before puberty, the squamocolumnar junction is inside the endocervical canal; (b) at puberty, cervical eversion occurs; (c) following puberty, the area of cervical ectopy becomes covered with squamous epithelium; (d) two squamocolumnar junctions result, and the area between them is the transformation zone; (e) after the menopause, the squamocolumnar junction formed following puberty ascends into the cervical canal.

Cervical ectopy is a physiological state stimulated by increased oestrogens; it can occur at puberty as described previously, but also occurs in women on the combined oral contraceptive pill and during pregnancy.

Cervical screening

In general terms, the purpose of a screening programme is to reduce the incidence of a specific cancer within a specified population. However, a number of conditions must exist in order to allow a screening programme to be implemented (Table 1.1). The only gynaecological malignancy that currently meets the screening criteria is cervical carcinoma. In 1952, Papanicolaou and Traut described a cervical smear technique capable of detecting abnormal cervical cytology suggestive of cervical dysplasia. Subsequent studies have shown that CIN is definitely a premalignant state and is the precursor of invasive squamous cervical carcinoma, not adenocarcinoma.

The use of colposcopy as an investigative technique was originally described by Hinsellman in 1926, but was not adopted as the investigation of choice for women with abnormal cervical cytology until the 1970s. Since then, the concept of local minimally invasive treatment has gained universal acceptance, and a 98% cure rate is possible.

Cervical cancer has been shown to be preventable, providing the design of the screening programme is appropriate. It has, however, been shown that increasing the frequency of screening beyond a certain level gives diminishing returns (Table 1.2), particularly in cost–benefit terms. The USA has implemented an annual screening programme, while the UK has a 3-yearly programme.

TABLE 1.1

Conditions conducive to the introduction of a screening programme

- Prolonged duration of premalignant state
- An effective (specific and sensitive) test to detect the premalignant phase
- Effective and readily available treatment for the premalignant state (preventing progression to malignancy)
- Demonstrable cost-effectiveness

TABLE 1.2

Detection rates for cervical screening* at varying screening intervals (%)

10-yearly	64
5-yearly	84
3-yearly	89
Annually	93.5

*Sexually active women are screened between the ages of 20 and 69 years

It is important to note that cervical cancer is associated with low socio-economic class; incidence is higher in precisely those women with least access to healthcare provision. It is, therefore, important that strenuous effort is made to access the whole population when implementing a screening programme.

Cervical smear interpretation has changed over the years and the original Papanicolaou classification has been simplified. In strict scientific terms, cytology should be reported in terms of dyskaryosis. However, to reduce confusion, laboratories report smear results as shown in Table 1.3. The diagnosis of CIN is only possible with histological confirmation, hence the emphasis on 'suggestive of'.

False-negative result. The Papanicolaou smear has been shown to have a false-negative rate in the range 5–50% (depending on the study quoted). A 5% false-negative smear rate has been accepted as actionable when smears are taken by well-trained healthcare professionals using colposcopic guidance, and are assessed by cytopathologists working to high standards of quality control. For smears taken without colposcopic guidance, the 'normal' false-negative rate is 10–20%. In the past, approximately half the errors in reported results were due to laboratory mistakes, and half occurred as a result of a poorly performed smear test. However, much stricter quality control in the laboratory means that the majority of false-negative results are now due to the clinician.

To minimize the sampling error and thus the cervical smear false-negative rate, smears must be taken with a spatula, with or without an endocervical

TABLE 1.3

Laboratory reporting of cervical smear interpretation

(a) Standard approach

Result	Action
Normal	Repeat as per national policy
Inflammatory	Screen for STDs. Repeat at 6 months
Suggestive of CIN 1	? colposcopy, ? repeat at 6 months
Suggestive of CIN 2	Refer for colposcopy
Suggestive of CIN 3	Refer for colposcopy
Suggestive of invasion	Refer for colposcopy, urgent

(b) New Bethesda classification

- Normal
- Inflammatory
- Atypical cells of undetermined significance
- Low-grade squamous cells (CIN 1)
- High-grade squamous cells (CIN 2, 3)

CIN = cervical intraepithelial neoplasia

brush, according to the type of cervix (Figure 1.2a–c). There are many varieties of spatula and the selected spatula should allow good contact with the transformation zone. Once taken, the sample should be promptly applied to the glass slide using a side-to-side motion (Figure 1.3) and fixed with alcohol to prevent air drying. The slide should be accurately pre-labelled, and sent to the laboratory in a shatterproof box. When followed diligently, these simple steps produce substantial improvement in the accuracy of the test. Recently, considerable effort has been devoted to improving the laboratory testing procedures, particularly using computerized screening methods to support laboratory personnel.

Colposcopy

Colposcopy is an investigative technique used for microscopic examination of the lower genital tract, including the cervix, vagina and vulva. The organs

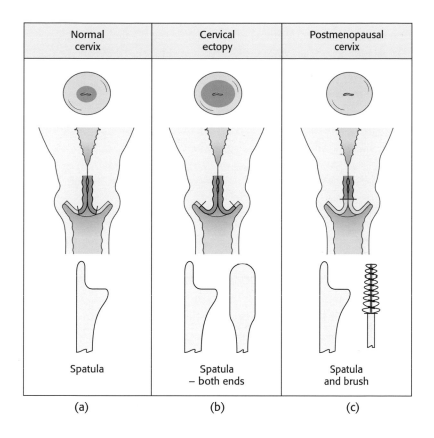

Normal cervix	Cervical ectopy	Postmenopausal cervix
Spatula	Spatula – both ends	Spatula and brush
(a)	(b)	(c)

Figure 1.2 Appropriate use of spatula and brush in cervical smear testing: (a) normal cervix; (b) cervical ectopy; (c) postmenopausal cervix.

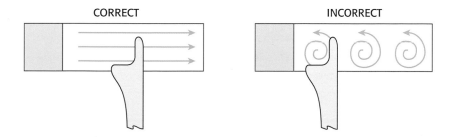

CORRECT

INCORRECT

Figure 1.3 Cervical smear being applied to a pre-labelled slide.

are viewed under magnifications of between 4- and 20-times normal.

On attendance at the colposcopy clinic, an abbreviated gynaecological history is taken and an explanation given to each patient. This should cover the following points:

- smears are designed to detect precancer not cancer
- the patient's doctor thought that her cervix looked normal (assuming he or she did) and therefore it is very unlikely that she has cancer
- CIN and its potential for malignant change over a long period of time if untreated
- colposcopy
- the available treatments
- 'see and treat' or 'wait for punch biopsy confirmation' before treatment.

The patient is placed in the lithotomy position and examined colposcopically. The colposcopist's approach varies but, in general, starts with a repetition of the cervical cytology under colposcopic guidance. Saline is then applied and the overall architecture of the cervix inspected. This is followed by application of acetic acid (3% or 5%) and the colposcopist looks for areas of aceto white (indicative of abnormal vascular pattern). Any such areas are biopsied and, finally, Lugol's iodine is applied; any areas failing to stain with the iodine are potentially abnormal.

The results of the colposcopy determine the next course of action. The algorithm in Figure 1.4 shows the various treatment options. Table 1.4 details treatments for CIN 3.

Treatment of cervical abnormality

Before out-patient treatments became available, cold-knife cone biopsy (removing the transformation zone to a depth of 2.5 cm) was both the investigation and the treatment of choice for cervical abnormality. A general anaesthetic was required, and the major disadvantage was that many women subsequently developed cervical incompetence or stenosis. This stimulated a search for less invasive procedures that could be performed under local anaesthetic without compromising child-bearing ability.

A more recent approach to the treatment of CIN is cryotherapy, which can be performed without anaesthetic. Its use should, however, be restricted to treatment of warts and possibly CIN 1. More recently still, laser treatment has been used either to ablate or to perform a 1 cm deep cervical

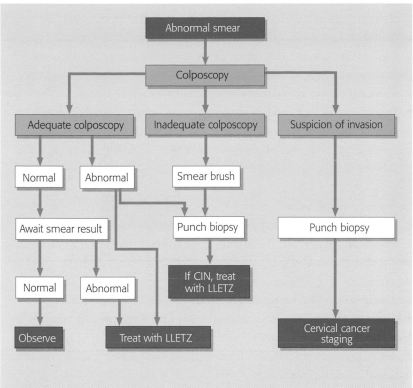

Figure 1.4 Treatment options following an abnormal smear.

TABLE 1.4

Treatments for CIN 3

Treatment	Efficacy	Anaesthesia	Cost of equipment	Tissue sample
Cryotherapy	80%	Local	< $2000	No
Cold coagulation	95–98%	Local	< $2000	No
Needle electrodiathermy	95–98%	General	< $100	No
Laser ablation	95–98%	Local	$70000	No
Laser conization	95–98%	Local	$70000	Yes
LLETZ	95–98%	Local	$2500	Yes

conization (Figure 1.5). Laser treatment now tends to be used only for vulval intraepithelial neoplasia (VIN) and vaginal intraepithelial neoplasia (VAIN).

Electrocautery is used by the majority of gynaecologists for excision of the transformation zone. This technique is commonly referred to as large loop excision of the transformation zone (LLETZ), and is now the dominant treatment method. The advantage of obtaining a tissue sample is that it may be sent for histological examination, making it much less likely that microinvasive carcinoma of the cervix will be accidentally ablated and the possibility of lymphatic disease spread missed.

Exclusion criteria. Some women who are excessively anxious about pelvic examination are unsuitable for either out-patient treatment or, rarely, for out-patient examination. These women should be investigated and treated under a general anaesthetic.

Follow up. After LLETZ treatment, patients should have a follow-up colposcopic examination and cervical smear at 4–6 months, and smears at 1 year and annually thereafter.

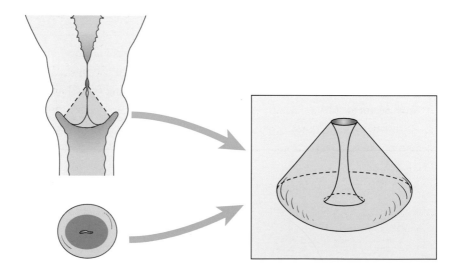

Figure 1.5 Local treatment of the transformation zone.

For women found to have invasive carcinoma, management guidelines are outlined on pages 18–22.

Cervical carcinoma staging

The staging of cervical carcinoma has, until recently, always been carried out pre-surgically. There is, however, currently much debate as to whether cervical carcinoma should be staged surgically, as pre-surgical staging can under- or overestimate the stage of disease (Table 1.5).

In general, a patient presenting with invasive carcinoma is referred to the colposcopy clinic because the physician taking a cervical smear recognizes that the cervix appears abnormal and makes an immediate referral. Occasionally, referral is made when the cervix looks macroscopically normal, but the smear is suggestive of malignancy. The patient may also be referred if the smear is suggestive of CIN 3 with a macroscopically normal cervix and, on colposcopy, a microinvasive tumour is detected. The final method of detection is where a woman develops symptoms (e.g. intermenstrual or postcoital bleeding) and is referred to the general gynaecology clinic where the disease is detected. This eventuality is, mercifully, becoming rarer due to the increasing effectiveness and reach of screening programmes.

In a patient with suspected cervical carcinoma, the disease requires a staging procedure that involves cystoscopy, colposcopy, vaginal examination, sigmoidoscopy and a rectal examination to assess the parametrium. This is carried out under general anaesthetic. Computed tomography (CT) scanning and magnetic resonance imaging (MRI) are usually performed to determine lymphadenopathy and parametrial spread respectively, although these are not technically included in the staging drawn up by the International Federation of Gynaecology and Obstetrics (FIGO staging; Figure 1.6).

Once histological confirmation has taken place and the tumour has been

TABLE 1.5

Staging of cervical cancer

	Overstage (%)	Understage (%)	Correct (%)
Stage Ib	14.5	19.0	66.5
Stage II	33.5	21.0	45.5

Figure 1.6 FIGO staging of cervical cancer.

Stage 0   Intraepithelial neoplasia

Stage I   The carcinoma is strictly confined to the cervix, extension to the uterine corpus should be disregarded

Ia   Preclinical carcinomas of the cervix (i.e. those diagnosed by microscopy only). All gross lesions even with superficial invasion are stage Ib. Invasion is limited to measured stromal invasion with a maximum depth of 5 mm and no wider than 7 mm. Measurement of the depth of invasion should be from the base of the epithelium, either surface or glandular, from which it originates. Vascular space involvement, either venous or lymphatic, should not alter the staging

Ia1   Minimal microscopically evident stromal invasion. The stromal invasion is no more than 3 mm deep and no more than 7 mm in diameter

Ia2   Lesions detected microscopically that can be measured. The measured invasion of the stroma is deeper than 3 mm but no greater than 5 mm, and the diameter is no wider than 7 mm

Ib   Clinical lesions confined to the cervix, or preclinical lesions greater than stage Ia

Ib1   Clinical lesions less than 4 cm in size

Ib2   Clinical lesions greater than 4 cm in size

Stage II   Involvement of the vagina except the lower third, or infiltration of the parametrium. No involvement of the pelvic sidewall

IIa   Involvement of the upper two-thirds of the vagina, but not out to the sidewall

IIb   Infiltration of the parametrium, but not out to the sidewall

Stage III   Involvement of the lower third of the vagina. Extension to the pelvic sidewall. On rectal examination there is no cancer-free space between the tumour and the pelvic sidewall. All cases with a hydronephrosis or non-functioning kidney should be included, unless this is known to be attributable to another cause

IIIa   Involvement of the lower third of the vagina, but not out to the pelvic sidewall if the parametrium is involved

IIIb   Extension onto the pelvic sidewall and/or hydronephrosis or non-functional kidney

Stage IV   Extension of the carcinoma beyond the reproductive tract

IVa   Involvement of the mucosa of the bladder or rectum

IVb   Distant metastasis or disease outside the true pelvis

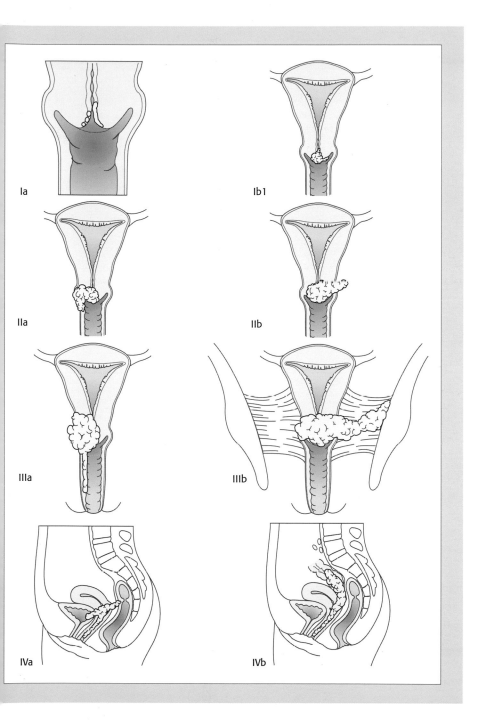

Ia

Ib1

IIa

IIb

IIIa

IIIb

IVa

IVb

staged, treatment can be planned. It should be remembered that any lack of concordance should lead to the more advanced stage being selected. The relatively poor sensitivity and specificity of clinical staging has led many to suggest that staging should be surgical.

Management

This depends primarily on the stage of the disease. For those women requiring a radical hysterectomy, the pre-operative investigation/ management (in addition to the staging procedure) should include:

- full blood cell count
- group and save/cross-match packed cells
- urea and electrolytes
- liver function tests
- CT, or preferably MRI, scanning
- chest X-ray
- electrocardiograph
- ureteric visualization (e.g. CT with contrast)
- prophylactic antibiotics
- thromboembolic prophylaxis: stockings and a heparin preparation.

Stage Ia1. This stage, defined as minimal microscopic invasion (< 3 mm), should be treated with local therapy in women wishing to retain their reproductive potential, assuming complete excision of the lesion is possible, with no lymphovascular permeation. In a woman past child-bearing age, many doctors in the USA might advise extrafascial (routine) hysterectomy.

Stage Ia2. Lesions with an invasion of greater than 3 mm, less than 5 mm in depth, and an area of less than 7 mm in width, with no lymphovascular permeation, can probably be treated effectively by conization, though radical trachelectomy/hysterectomy may be warranted. For these lesions, treatment should be individualized; those patients not wishing to retain their fertility will undergo radical hysterectomy and pelvic lymphadenectomy, as described overleaf. For those wishing to retain fertility, a cone biopsy may be performed if there is an absence of lymphovascular permeation. If there is suspicion of lymph involvement, laparoscopic lymph node sampling and radical trachelectomy may be the treatment methods of choice.

Radical hysterectomy for stage Ia2 cervical cancer involves removal of the cervix, uterus, upper third of vagina, the parametrium, and the external, internal and obturator nodes. The para-aortic and common iliac nodes may also be removed. With large tumours, pretreatment with chemotherapy may be beneficial; this is currently being investigated.

Women with positive nodes should be given further therapy with external beam radiotherapy. The value of adjuvant chemotherapy is currently being assessed in trials.

Stage Ib (Ib1< 4 cm in diameter; Ib2 > 4 cm in diameter). The management of this stage is primarily surgical and should comprise a radical hysterectomy, with or without ovarian conservation (depending on age).

Stage IIa. Treatment depends on the centre involved. Many will undertake radical surgery with similar criteria for adjuvant therapy, as with stage Ib. Some centres will not perform surgery, but will use radiotherapy administered by intracavity and external beam radiation.

Stage IIb. Until recently, management has exclusively involved radiotherapy with no surgery. Trials are, however, currently under way to assess pretreatment with chemotherapy, with a view to 'downstaging' the disease so that it involves the cervix alone, thereby permitting surgery. In addition, a few surgeons are commencing primary treatment with surgery. Those patients who do undergo surgery also receive adjuvant radiotherapy or chemotherapy.

Stages IIIa, IIIb and IV. Treatment is with radiotherapy. Trials with adjuvant chemotherapy are currently under way.

Surgery

Radical hysterectomy involves the removal of the uterine body, cervix, upper third of the vagina, parametrium, the paracervical, obturator, internal, external, and common iliac nodes plus or minus the para-aortic nodes (Figure 1.7). It can be performed using either a mid-line or a modified Cherny's low transverse incision.

For patients wishing to preserve fertility, laparoscopic lymphadenectomy

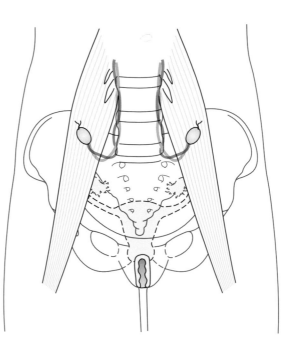

Figure 1.7 Radical hysterectomy showing removal of uterus, cervix, parametrium, upper third vagina and lymph nodes. The ovaries are attached to the source muscle intra-abdominally.

can be performed, coupled with a vaginal approach to remove the cervix, known as radical trachelectomy (Figure 1.8). Alternatively, radical trachelectomy may be performed via an abdominal route. These procedures, particularly radical trachelectomy, should still be regarded as experimental, but should be discussed with young women without children.

Radiotherapy

When given as an adjunct to surgery, radiotherapy is administered using an external beam source. When radiotherapy is the sole treatment, it is also given by intracavity radiotherapy and external beam. Intracavity radiotherapy involves insertion of radioactive material high into the vagina. The procedure is not painful. It is important that appropriate dosing is administered to the central tumour and the pelvic sidewall nodes. Dose is usually calculated at radiotherapy points known as A and B. Point A is situated 2 cm from the mid-line of the cervical canal and is used relative to the central tumour, while point B is 3 cm to the side of point A (Figure 1.9). Point B and the overlying tissue are important relative to nodal tissue.

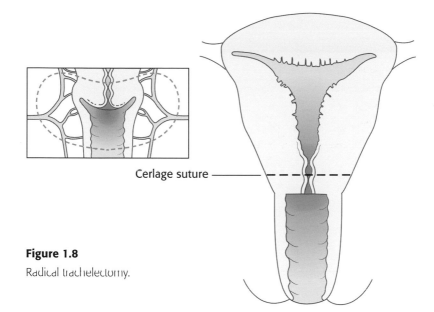

Cerlage suture ————

Figure 1.8
Radical trachelectomy.

Prognosis

A patient's prognosis is determined by stage, nodal status and tumour type. An overview of the prognosis according to cancer stage is shown in Table 1.6. In general, cervical squamous carcinoma has a better prognosis than adenosquamous carcinoma, stage for stage. In addition, adenocarcinoma tends to be diagnosed later, and therefore at a more advanced stage, thus worsening the prognosis.

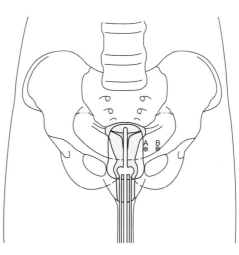

Figure 1.9 Points A and B as used in radiotherapy.

TABLE 1.6

5-year cure rates in cervical carcinoma

Stage	Cure rate (%)
I	91
IIa	83
IIb	66
IIIa	45
IIIb	36
IV	14

Vaginal carcinoma

Primary vaginal carcinomas are rare. A vaginal tumour is usually secondary to cervical carcinoma (stage IIa, IIIa).

CHAPTER 2

Endometrial cancer

Epidemiology

Adenocarcinoma of the endometrium is the most common gynaecological malignancy, and the fourth most common malignancy in women. In the USA, over 30 000 women develop endometrial cancer annually, making it one and a half times as common as ovarian carcinoma, and three times as common as cervical cancer.

The incidence of endometrial cancer appears to have increased during the 1970s and 1980s, but the predicted death rate has fallen. Both the rise in incidence and the fall in the death rate may be due to the increase in the use of hormone replacement therapy and the associated ascertainment of disease at an earlier stage. Endometrial carcinoma occurs pre- and postmenopausally. The median age of patients is 61 years, and most are between 50 and 59 years. Approximately 5% of patients will be diagnosed before the age of 40, and 20–25% will be diagnosed before the menopause. Use of the oral contraceptive pill and cigarette smoking appear to reduce the risk of endometrial cancer, whilst obesity, nulliparity and late menopause increase risk (Table 2.1).

Pathology

Histologically, endometrial carcinoma falls into the following subtypes:
- adenocarcinoma (60%)
- adenoacanthoma (22%)
- adenosquamous carcinoma (7%)
- clear-cell carcinoma (6%)
- papillary adenocarcinoma (4%)
- secretory carcinoma (1%).

Carcinoma of the corpus should be graded according to the degree of differentiation of the adenocarcinoma, as shown below.
- G1: < 5% nonsquamous or nonmorular solid growth pattern
- G2: 6–50% nonsquamous or nonmorular solid growth pattern
- G3: > 50% nonsquamous or nonmorular solid growth pattern.

In most large series, 75% of patients are diagnosed as stage I, 11% stage II, 11% stage III, and 3% stage IV.

TABLE 2.1

Risk factors for endometrial carcinoma

Factor	Risk ratio
Combined oral contraceptive pill	0.5
Smoking	0.7
Obesity	
overweight by 20–50 lb	3
overweight by > 50 lb	10
Nulliparity	
compared with +1 child	2
compared with +5 children	3
Late menopause	
age > 52 years versus < 49 years	2.4
Unopposed oestrogen replacement therapy without a progestational agent	6.0
Diabetes mellitus	2.7
Tamoxifen	2.2

(Modified from DiSaia and Creasman, 1993)

Diagnosis

Currently, it is not possible to rationalize a population-based screening programme for endometrial cancer. In the postmenopausal woman, the disease usually presents as postmenopausal bleeding. In the premenopausal woman, it presents as menstrual irregularity with irregular or heavy vaginal bleeding. Approximately 20% of women with endometrial carcinoma are diagnosed as a result of abnormal endometrial cells seen on cervical smear. The smear is not, however, an appropriate method for routine detection of endometrial cancer. Postmenopausal bleeding must always be investigated by endometrial sampling. Traditionally, this took the form of a dilatation and curettage (D & C) operation carried out under either a general anaesthetic or intravenous analgesia and paracervical block.

Nowadays, sampling tends to be performed either with an endometrial aspirator (Figure 2.1) plus an ultrasound scan for endometrial thickness, or by hysteroscopy with a biopsy (Figure 2.2). Once histological diagnosis has been made, the patient will usually be admitted for surgical management. Since 1988, endometrial cancer has been staged surgically (Figure 2.3). For a patient who is too frail to withstand surgery, radiotherapy may be used as the first-line therapy. However, for most patients, the cancer can be accurately staged surgically.

Pre-operative investigations

All patients should receive the following pre-operative investigation and management:

- full blood count
- urea and electrolytes
- liver function tests
- chest X-ray
- CT/MRI scan of the abdomen and pelvis
- electrocardiograph
- group and save/cross match blood
- thromboembolic and antibiotic prophylaxis.

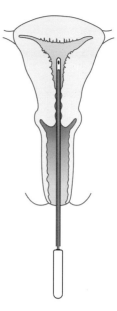

Figure 2.1 Sampling with endometrial aspirator.

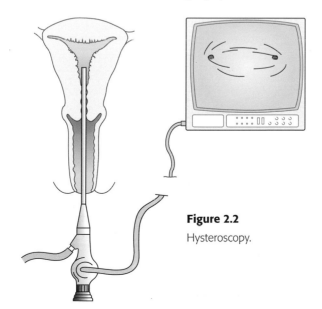

Figure 2.2
Hysteroscopy.

Figure 2.3 FIGO staging of endometrial carcinoma.

Stage I

Ia G1,2,3   Tumour limited to the endometrium

Ib G1,2,3   Invasion of less than half of the myometrium

Ic G1,2,3   Invasion of more than half of the myometrium

Stage II

IIa G1,2,3   Endocervical glandular involvement only

IIb G1,2,3   Cervical stromal invasion

Stage III

IIIa G1,2,3   Tumour invades serosa and/or adenexae and/or malignant
                     peritoneal cytology

IIIb G1,2,3   Vaginal metastases

IIIc G1,2,3   Metastases to pelvic and/or para-aortic lymph nodes

Stage IV

IVa G1,2,3   Tumour invasion of the bladder and/or bowel mucosa

IVb   Distant metastases including intra-abdominal and/or inguinal
                    lymph nodes

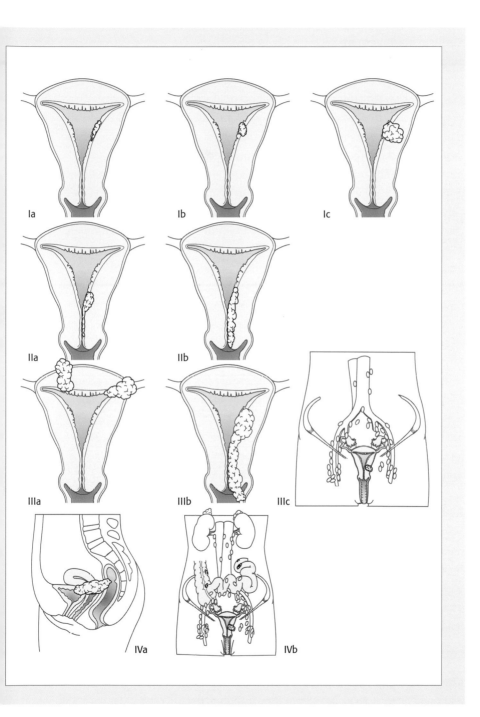

Surgical management

Surgical management of endometrial carcinoma, specifically the ideal degree of radicality (i.e. radical hysterectomy and lymphadenectomy versus routine extrafascial hysterectomy) required for optimal treatment, has been extensively debated over the last few years. Discussion is clouded by the fact that many of the patients are high risk from both a surgical and anaesthetic viewpoint because they are, for example, elderly, overweight, diabetic or hypertensive. The minimum that should be undertaken is an extrafascial (total) abdominal hysterectomy with full examination of the abdomen and pelvis; washings and diaphragmatic smears should also be taken for cytology. In addition, omentectomy should ideally be performed, although some patients may be deemed unsuitable for a mid-line incision. Furthermore, some gynaecologists perform pelvic and para-aortic lymphadenectomy, others carry out general lymph node sampling or sample only suspicious nodes. Some specialists do not sample lymph nodes at all. US practice veers more towards lymphadenectomy than UK practice.

Nodal sampling results in upward staging in many patients with myometrial invasion. The surgical staging protocol is shown in Table 2.2.

Postoperatively, decisions about further therapy depend on the stage of the tumour and its histological grade. For women with stage I G1 tumours there is agreement that hysterectomy and bilateral salpingo-oophorectomy are the only treatments required. It may be that surgery alone is adequate for all surgically staged stage I lesions, but most doctors would give radiotherapy to patients with G3 lesions and stage Ic lesions.

Radiotherapy

When radiotherapy is given after surgery, it is external beam with a view to eradicating possible micrometastases to the pelvic lymph nodes. Pre-operative radiotherapy can be given in varying pre-surgical doses to women with larger uteri. The time that radiotherapy is given before surgery depends on the size of the uterus. There is general agreement that surgery alone is inadequate for patients with stage II or more advanced cancer, and adjuvant radiotherapy is required.

Chemotherapy

Although progestogens have been used as adjunctive therapy in endometrial

TABLE 2.2

Surgical staging sheet for endometrial/ovarian carcinoma

Incision:	Low transverse	mid-line	paramedian
		Histology	
Findings:	Uterus		
	Tubes		
	Ovaries		
	Omentum		
Nodes:	External iliac		
	Internal iliac		
	Obturator		
	Common iliac		
	Para-aortic		
	Peritoneal surfaces		
	Peritoneal washings		

Description of operation:

Stage:

cancer for over 20 years, there are now numerous studies that demonstrate their lack of efficacy. Some patients with recurrent disease do, however, benefit from progestogen treatment. Patients likely to benefit are those with grade 1 tumours that have oestrogen and progestogen receptors. About one-third of patients with recurrence will respond to progestogen treatment. The preferred dosing schedule is either 500 mg medroxyprogesterone acetate (Depo-Provera®) intramuscularly at weekly intervals, or oral medroxyprogesterone acetate (Provera®), 200 mg daily. Recurrent disease has also been shown to respond to other chemotherapeutic agents (e.g. cisplatin). As with other gynaecological tumours, long-term follow up is necessary. Traditionally, this involves pelvic examination and vaginal vault cytology. However, there is increasing evidence that follow up with pelvic examination alone is adequate.

TABLE 2.3

Risk of recurrence in women with endometrial cancer

Low risk

Stage I, G1,2, non-serous and non-clear-cell adenocarcinoma with invasion of the inner third or less of the myometrium

Intermediate risk

Stage I, G1,2,3, non-serous and non-clear-cell adenocarcinoma with invasion of the middle or deep third of the myometrium

High risk

Stage II, III or IV disease, serous or clear-cell carcinoma

Prognosis

The prognosis of patients with endometrial cancer is related to the stage of the disease and the histological grade of the tumour. It is, therefore, related to the depth of myometrial invasion, the degree of involvement of the lymph nodes, the adnexa, and the presence of positive peritoneal washings. Table 2.3 classifies the risk of recurrence as low, intermediate or high. In addition, the prognosis is related to tumour receptor status and the DNA ploidy of the tumour. Survival rates at 5 years are 72% for stage I, 56% for stage II, 31% for stage III, and 10% for stage IV.

CHAPTER 3

Ovarian cancer

Epidemiology

In terms of mortality, ovarian cancer is the most common cancer affecting the female genital tract. Overall, lymphomas and cancers of the breast, colon and uterus are more common than ovarian cancer. Cancer of the ovary is the second most common gynaecological cancer, accounting for 26% of tumours, but 52% of the total mortality. The probability of a newborn female developing ovarian cancer over the course of her lifetime is 1.4% (i.e. 1 in 70).

Ovarian cancer is most common in women aged 55–59 years, but can occur at any age. Incidence is higher among white women than black women, and is increasing. The associated death rate has doubled over the past 40 years. This is in contrast to the incidence of breast cancer, which has remained constant, and cervical and endometrial cancers which have fallen in incidence. The trend in incidence is probably due to women having smaller families and, with increasing affluence, an increasingly high-fat diet.

A number of epidemiological risk factors are associated with ovarian cancer. These include nulliparity, infertility, marked premenstrual tension, a high-fat diet, higher socio-economic status, family history, celibacy, increased number of abortions, irradiation of pelvic organs, early menopause, type Λ blood, and exposure to talcs and asbestos. There is also an association with breast and endometrial cancer, and all three cancers are associated with high-fat diets. An association has also recently been reported between exposure to ovarian stimulatory drugs and ovarian cancer. This finding is consistent with the observation that factors that suppress ovulation (e.g. pregnancy and the oral contraceptive pill) are protective.

Screening

Much effort is currently being made to develop a screening test for ovarian cancer. Unfortunately, most ovarian tumours present at an advanced stage, with the result that survival rates are poor. The search for an effective screening test has been hampered by uncertainty over whether a premalignant phase of the disease can be detected. Any test must have a very high specificity and sensitivity because of the difficulty in evaluating the ovaries.

To date, research has centred around vaginal examination, ultrasound scanning (including colour flow Doppler imaging), and the use of tumour markers, the most promising of which is Ca 125. However, currently none of these techniques, either alone or in combination, has proved suitable for screening the general population. The relative specificities and sensitivities of each test are shown in Table 3.1.

The search continues for a suitable screening test. In the UK, a study is currently under way using a combination of vaginal examination, Doppler ultrasound and tumour markers. The investigators expect to recruit 20 000 women. The results of this study may make screening a practical proposition, at least for postmenopausal women.

It is known that ovarian cancer is genetically heritable. In the UK and the USA, screening using Ca 125 and ultrasound is now recommended for those women with two first-degree relatives diagnosed as having ovarian cancer. Risk of developing cancer based on familial incidence has also been defined by Lynch (Table 3.2). The work of Lynch and others, based on gynaecological studies of families, has demonstrated that there is a 'cancer-prone' family. Members of this family have an increased risk of developing carcinoma of breast, colon, ovaries and endometrium.

Genetic testing is beyond the scope of this text.

TABLE 3.1

Potential tests for detecting early stage ovarian cancer

Test	Specificity (%)	Sensitivity at 1 year (%)
Ca 125	97.0	70
Vaginal examination	97.3	–
Ultrasound	98.0	90
Vaginal examination and ultrasound	99.0	–
Ca 125 and ultrasound	99.8	70
Ca 125 and vaginal examination	100	70
Ca 125, ultrasound and vaginal examination	100	–

TABLE 3.2

Risk of heritable ovarian cancer

Number of first-degree relatives affected	Relative risk
One	2.5
Two	30

Pathology

In 1973, WHO guidelines on the histological classification of ovarian malignancy were published; the broad divisions are shown in Table 3.3. The classification differentiates epithelial tumours into benign, borderline and malignant grades, and according to whether adenomatous or fibrous elements are dominant.

A borderline tumour has some but not all of the features of cancer including, in varying combinations:

- stratification of the epithelial cells
- apparent detachment of cellular clusters from their sites of origin
- mitotic activity
- nuclear abnormalities intermediate between those of clearly benign or malignant changes.

Obvious stromal invasion must not be present in tumours classified as borderline.

Staging

Staging of ovarian cancer can only be carried out surgically, and it is vitally important that a complete staging procedure is always undertaken. Inadequate staging, followed at a later date by adequate staging, has demonstrated that approximately 30% of women are more advanced than originally thought. Laparotomy should take place through a mid-line vertical incision. The staging procedure is similar to that for endometrial cancer (Table 2.2, page 29). The FIGO staging for ovarian cancer is shown in Figure 3.1. Tumours are also graded and the gradation affects both prognosis and treatment of the patient.

TABLE 3.3

Histological classification of ovarian malignancies

I   Common epithelial tumours

(Each type is classified as benign, borderline, malignant)

A   Serous

B   Mucinous

C   Endometrioid

D   Clear cell (mesonephroid)

E   Brenner tumours

F   Mixed epithelial tumours

G   Undifferentiated carcinoma

H   Unclassified epithelial tumours

II Sex cord (gonadal stromal) tumours

A   Granulosa–stromal cell tumour

B   Androblastoma; Sertoli–Leydig cell tumour

C   Gynandroblastoma

D   Unclassified

III Lipid (lipoid) cell tumours

IV Germ cell tumours

A   Dysgerminoma

B   Endodermal sinus tumour

C   Embryonal carcinoma

D   Polyembryoma

E   Choriocarcinoma

F   Teratoma

G   Mixed forms

Management

Pre-operative investigations. The problems associated with making a suspected diagnosis pre-operatively are similar to those of investigation prior to surgery. They are due to an inability to visualize accurately the extent of pathology using current imaging techniques.

Ultrasound is a good technique for detecting ovarian cysts, particularly when augmented with Doppler colour flow imaging. It is, however, a poor tool for visualizing nodal disease and peritoneal involvement. CT scanning gives better visualization of lymph nodes, but will only detect nodes greater than 1 cm in diameter. CT scanning can also detect liver metastases, ascites and peritoneal involvement, though it is not uncommon for these to be under- or overdiagnosed. MRI scanning may provide a useful adjunct, but is subject to similar errors. CT is probably still the best modality for identifying lymph nodes, whereas MRI has the edge in assessing soft tissue spread.

Every patient should have the following pre-operative investigation/management:

- full blood count
- group and save/cross-match packed cells
- urea and electrolytes
- liver function tests
- Ca 125
- carcinoembryonic antigen (CEA)
- serum stored for other tumour markers if required
- pelvic examination and cervical smear
- CT scan
- ultrasound scan
- bowel preparation (in case colostomy is required)
- antibiotic and thromboprophylaxis.

Before surgery, extensive discussion with the patient is required, based partly on the results of the preparatory investigations. Unfortunately, with ovarian cancer, it is not possible to predict accurately the stage of disease before laparotomy. In a postmenopausal woman with an adnexal mass, it is standard procedure to carry out a hysterectomy, bilateral salpingo-oophorectomy, and greater omentectomy. In addition, lymphadenectomy or sampling may be performed, as may bowel resection if the bowel is involved.

Figure 3.1 FIGO staging of ovarian cancer.

Stage I   Growth limited to the ovaries

Ia   Growth limited to one ovary, no ascites

Ia1   No tumour on the external surface, capsule intact

Ia2   Tumour present on the external surface and/or capsule ruptured

Ib   Growth limited to both ovaries, no ascites

Ib1   No tumour on the external surface, capsule intact

Ib2   Tumour present on the external surface and/or capsule ruptured

Ic   Tumour either stage Ia or b but with ascites or positive peritoneal washings

Stage II   Growth involving one or both ovaries with pelvic extension

IIa   Extension and/or metastases to the uterus and/or tubes

IIb   Extension to other pelvic tissues

IIc   Tumour either stage IIa or b, but with ascites or positive peritoneal washings

Stage III   Growth involving one or both ovaries with intraperitoneal metastases outside the pelvis and/or positive retroperitoneal or inguinal nodes; or tumour limited to the true pelvis with histologically proven malignant extension to small bowel or omentum; superficial liver metastases equals stage III

IIIa   Tumour grossly limited to the true pelvis with negative nodes but with histologically confirmed microscopic seeding of abdominal peritoneal surfaces

IIIb   Tumour of one or both ovaries; histologically confirmed implants of abdominal peritoneal surfaces, none exceeding 2 cm in diameter; nodes negative

IIIc   Abdominal implants 2 cm in diameter and/or positive retroperitoneal nodes or inguinal nodes

Stage IV   Growth involving one or both ovaries with distant metastases. If pleural effusion is present, there must be positive cytology to allot a patient to stage IV. Parenchymal liver metastases equal stage IV

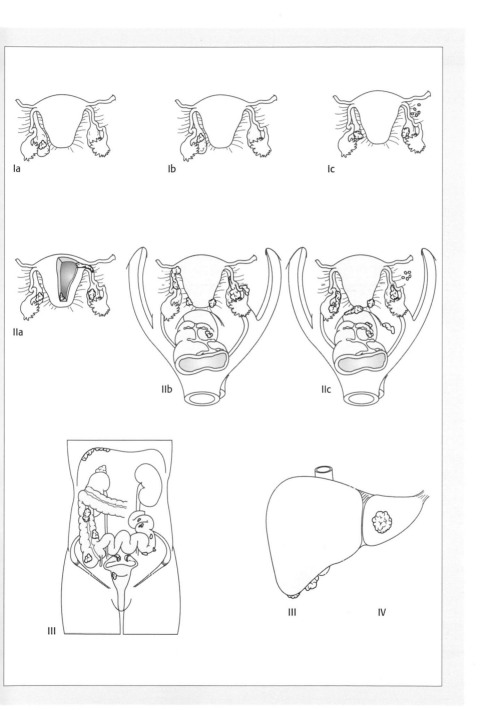

Ia

Ib

Ic

IIa

IIb

IIc

III

III

IV

Management of a premenopausal woman wishing to retain her fertility has to be highly individualized and based on the intra-operative findings. Many women opt to have an oophorectomy and full surgical staging, with the possibility of a further laparotomy to remove the other ovary and the uterus if required.

Differentiation between benign and malignant disease is often not possible either at laparotomy or on frozen section, and diagnosis must be confirmed by histology. In some patients, malignancy is more obvious, but even here pseudomyxoma can masquerade as malignancy. Therefore, if in doubt, the gynaecological oncologist should always wait for full histology results. When invasive disease is confirmed, management of the disease must comprise unilateral/bilateral oophorectomy and omentectomy with or without hysterectomy/bowel resection proportional to organ involvement.

For the patient, however, terrible uncertainty exists until after the operation. Careful and extensive pre-operative counselling is, therefore, mandatory for all patients.

Intra-operative management. The absolute minimum level of investigation is peritoneal washings, and diaphragmatic and paracolic gutter smears for cytology. In addition, the affected ovary should be removed and greater omentectomy should be performed. Suspicious peritoneal lesions should be biopsied and sent for histological investigation. Any palpable lymph nodes should be sampled and many gynaecological oncologists advocate complete lymphadenectomy.

Surgery aims to reduce tumour cell volume as much as possible. The ideal outcome is that no macroscopic tumour is visible at the end of the procedure. Failing this, the tumour should be reduced to nodules of less than 2 cm and preferably less than 1 cm. 'Heroic' surgery that is unlikely to reduce the tumour to at least less than 2 cm in diameter is probably best avoided as survival appears to be dependent on reaching this level.

Postoperative treatment. The majority of patients will have cancer in stages II, III and IV. Stages Ia and Ib are manageable by surgery alone, but those patients who are stages Ia with spillage, Ib with spillage, Ic, II, III or IV require adjuvant chemotherapy. Postoperative management of stage Ia (grade 3) and Ib differs between the UK and USA; adjuvant chemotherapy is usually used in the USA, while in the UK, most patients are managed individually and on an expectant basis. A UK study is currently under way that is addressing the need for chemotherapy in stage Ia tumours with spillage.

Repeat, or 'second-look' laparotomy after chemotherapy was a standard regimen in the late 1970s and 1980s, though the approach was adopted without rigorous evaluation. It is now used in many trial protocols and there is some evidence that there may be benefit in operating after chemotherapy has been used to achieve tumour shrinkage.

Patients without evidence of persistent disease following chemotherapy, and after tumour marker assessment and an MRI/CT scan, may benefit from laparoscopy and peritoneal lavage, with biopsy of any lesion.

Chemotherapy. There have been many advances in this field over the last 20 years. Of these, the three most significant have been the introduction of:

- alkylating agents – 1970s
- platinum-based agents (which extended median survival from 12 to 20 months) – 1980s
- paclitaxel in combination therapy, further extending median survival to 36 months – 1990s.

Compelling evidence now exists to support the use of paclitaxel combined with cis-platinum in the management of advanced (stages III and IV) ovarian cancer. This treatment regimen has been shown to be superior to previous treatments for tumours that have been debulked optimally (< 2 cm) and suboptimally (> 2 cm), in terms of progression-free survival and quality of life. Overall, this combination probably contributes, on average, an extra year of life at a cost of £7200 per life-year gained. Response to second-line treatment in patients who have relapsed following first-line treatment depends on the length of the initial remission period – the longer the remission, the better the prognosis.

Further developments, including high-dose chemotherapy and intraperitoneal therapy, are on the horizon. There are data that suggest that intraperitoneal therapy and high-dose chemotherapy improve survival times of patients with ovarian cancer who have not responded to, or have relapsed following standard therapeutic regimens. Currently these data are not sufficient to evaluate rigorously either improved survival times or a reduction in mortality resulting from these treatment methods. As with all

TABLE 3.4

Survival rates in patients with ovarian cancer

Stage	3-year survival rate (%)	5-year survival rate (%)
I	79.8	72.8
II	60.5	46.3
III	26.0	17.2
IIIa	41.7	30.7
IIIb	39.3	31.7
IIIc	22.3	14.4
IV	10.1	4.8
No stage	31.7	21.6
Total	43.4	34.9

Adapted from Pettersson, 1988

new therapeutic regimens, only appropriately designed, longitudinal studies of sufficient sample size have any chance of statistically demonstrating effects on these indices or coming to any clinically meaningful conclusions.

Prognosis

Prognosis in patients with ovarian cancer depends on the stage of the tumour (Table 3.4) and the efficacy of the debulking procedure. If no grossly visible residual tumour is left after surgery, 81% of patients will be in remission at second-look laparotomy, while 52% of patients left with optimal residual tumour mass (< 2 cm) will be in remission at follow up. In contrast, suboptimal debulking (> 2 cm) results in only 23% of patients remaining clear of disease.

Whatever the surgical outcome, treatment with first-line cis-platinum and paclitaxel has been shown to improve prognosis.

Cancer of the Fallopian tubes

Cancer of the Fallopian tubes is rare, and is often mistaken for ovarian cancer until laparotomy is performed. The tumour is staged surgically, and the procedure is similar to that used to stage ovarian malignancy (Table 2.2, page 29). Further discussion is outside the scope of this text.

CHAPTER 4

Vulval cancer

Epidemiology and aetiology

Vulval cancer accounts for 3–5% of all genital tract malignancies in women and its incidence appears to be increasing. It is primarily a disease of the elderly. In many series, over half of patients are over the age of 70 years, and the rising incidence of vulval cancer may therefore reflect the ageing female population. However, it has also been noted that approximately 15% of women with vulval cancer are under 40 years old. The aetiology is not as well understood as cervical neoplasia, but sexually transmitted diseases (STDs) appear to be involved. An association between HPV and vulval cancer has been shown, but no cause and effect has been proven. Ulcerative genital disease may also be associated with vulval neoplasia.

Pathology

Most lesions are squamous (85%) in origin (Figure 4.1), but all cancers that can affect skin can also affect the vulva. These include melanoma, sarcoma, adenocarcinoma and basal cell carcinoma. In addition, tumours can arise in Bartholin's glands (1%).

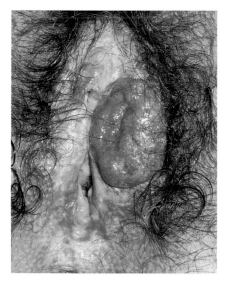

Figure 4.1 Exophytic squamous vulval carcinoma involving left labial minor and majoria; 4 x 5 cm in size.

Staging

The staging of vulval carcinoma has changed greatly over the years and many different classifications have been used. Modern staging uses the tumour–node–metastasis (TNM) classification and is based on surgical rather than clinical findings (Figure 4.2, pages 44–5).

Management

Clinical presentation. Lesions probably develop, over a prolonged period of time, from vulval intraepithelial neoplasia (VIN). VIN may be asymptomatic or may be associated with pruritus. Many lesions arise *de novo*. Wart-like growth may occur, and this may be confused with condyloma acuminatum. Patients with frank carcinoma may have either cauliflower-like growth or ulceration. These may be asymptomatic or associated with pruritus, pain, bleeding and a foul smell. On questioning, many patients will admit to having symptoms over many months and, unfortunately, many patients may also have been treated medically without biopsy for many months before referral for biopsy. The golden rule with vulval lesions is: always carry out a biopsy.

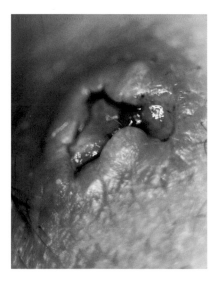

Figure 4.3 An herpetic ulcer on a background of HIV infection. Clinically, this was highly suspicious of carcinoma.

Any ulcerative lesion suspected of having an infectious aetiology (Figure 4.3) should be investigated thoroughly by an STD specialist. If tests are negative or the lesion does not respond promptly to medical management, a biopsy should be performed. Similarly, any growths on the vulva should be biopsied. If vulval warts are being treated with ablative therapy, it is important that there should be follow up to confirm that they have disappeared. Again, if they do not disappear, biopsy should be performed. If there is any suspicion that a lesion may be more than a wart, biopsy should take place prior to ablation. Rarely, syphilis may present in the secondary phase with condylomata (Figure 4.4).

Pre-operative investigations. The size of the lesion, the status of lymph nodes (determined clinically) and a biopsy should be performed on each patient to determine the depth of the tumour invasion. A CT scan may also be useful to determine the status of the lymph nodes, though no investigation is yet reliable enough to eliminate the need for lymphadenectomy except in the earliest cases of tumour invasion.

Early-stage vulval tumours with invasion less than 1 mm may be managed using conservative surgery, with wide local excision. In cases of deeper invasion, partial or two-stage lymphadenectomy may be performed (Figure 4.5). This is particularly important for younger patients, for whom the extremely mutilating effects of radical vulvectomy and lymphadenectomy are the most disturbing.

Although many patients are elderly and represent a poor anaesthetic risk, patients with vulval cancer should be managed surgically if at all possible. This type of tumour is resistant to both chemotherapy and radiotherapy, and failure to excise the tumour leaves the patient with a painful, slow and lingering demise. Pre-operative investigations/management should include:

- full blood count
- urea and electrolytes
- liver function tests
- cross-match packed cells/group and save
- CT/MRI scan
- chest X-ray
- electrocardiograph
- pelvic examination and Papanicolaou smear
- psychosexual counselling
- thromboembolic and antibiotic prophylaxis.

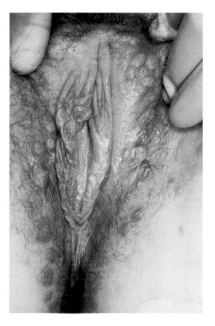

Figure 4.4 Secondary syphilis showing condylomata.

Figure 4.2 Tumour–node–metastasis (TNM) staging of vulval carcinoma.

Stage 0   Carcinoma *in situ*, intraepithelial carcinoma

Stage I   Lesions of 2 cm or less confined to the vulva or perineum. Absence of lymph node metastases

Ia   Lesions of 2 cm or less in size, confined to the vulva or perineum with stromal invasion to a depth of no more than 1 mm. No nodal metastases

Ib   Lesions of 2 cm or less in size, confined to the vulva or perineum with stromal invasion to a depth greater than 1 mm

Stage II   Tumour confined to the vulva and/or perineum, or more than 2 cm at its greatest dimension. No nodal metastases

Stage III   Tumour of any size on the vulva and/or perineum with:

(1) adjacent spread to the lower urethra and/or the vagina or the anus

and/or

(2) unilateral regional lymph node metastases

Stage IV

IVa   Tumour invading any of the following: upper urethra, bladder mucosa, rectal mucosa, pelvic bone, and/or bilateral regional node metastases

IVb   Any distant metastases including pelvic lymph nodes

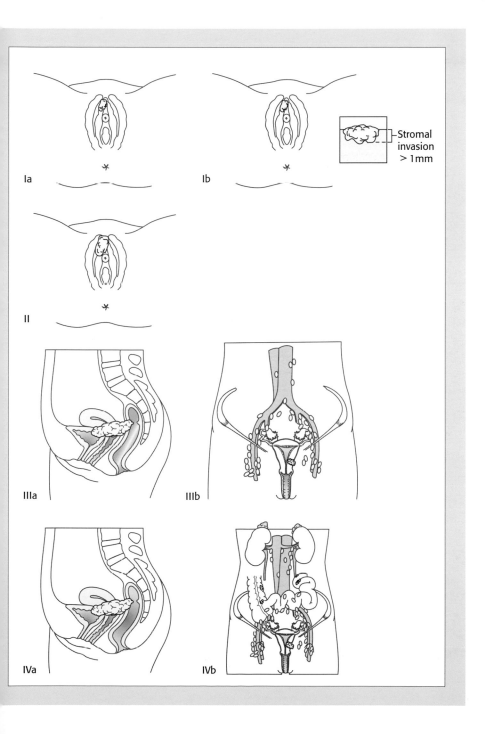

Ia

Ib

Stromal invasion >1mm

II

IIIa

IIIb

IVa

IVb

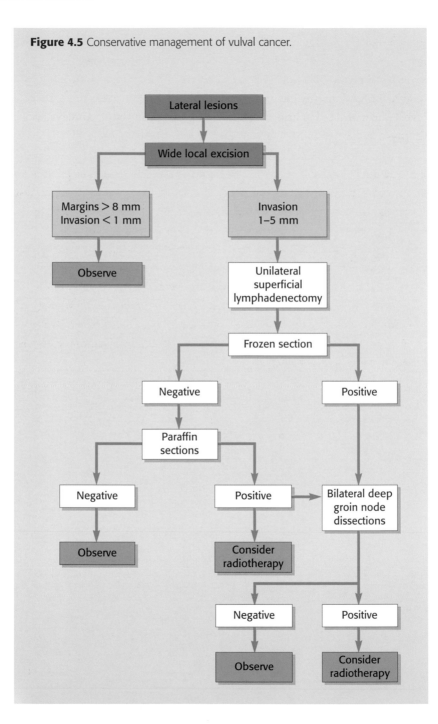

Figure 4.5 Conservative management of vulval cancer.

Intra-operative management. The standard management for lesions that are invasive to a depth of more than 5 mm is radical vulvectomy and removal of inguinal and femoral nodes. This is usually carried out via separate incisions (Figure 4.6). A butterfly incision is now rarely necessary, unless there is involvement of the skin bridge. As described previously, more conservative therapy may be possible for less invasive lesions.

Postoperative treatment. The most common postoperative complication is wound breakdown, which requires a prolonged stay in hospital. Lymphocyst formation in the groin is another problem, but this can be prevented using suction drainage. Approximately 5–10% of patients will develop lymphoedema in one or both lower limbs; the use of stockings for the first year postoperatively is helpful, as is prophylaxis with low-dose antibiotics.

No further treatment may be required after complete excision of the tumour if the lymph nodes are not involved. Long-term follow up by examination and cytology is still mandatory. For those patients with lymph node involvement, external beam radiotherapy should be given to the groins in case of microscopic metastases.

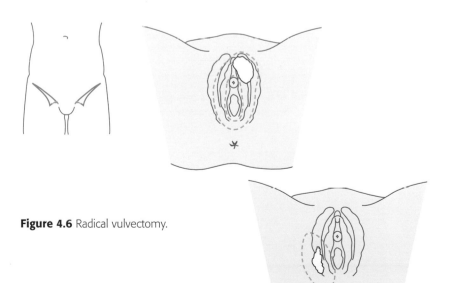

Figure 4.6 Radical vulvectomy.

Prognosis

In patients with vulval cancer, prognosis is partly determined by the age of the patient, and because initial diagnosis occurs most frequently in women over 70 years old, corrected 5-year survival rates should be quoted. For patients with stage I and II disease, 5-year survival rates of over 90% are to be expected if nodes are not involved. Nodal involvement reduces the 5-year survival rate to approximately 30%, though this is dependent on the number of nodes involved and whether or not the involvement is bilateral.

Cancer of the urethra

A primary tumour in this area is rare. Urethral carcinoma is usually secondary to vulval carcinoma (stages III and IV).

CHAPTER 5
Gestational trophoblastic neoplasia

Gestational trophoblastic neoplasia (GTN) is the term applied to choriocarcinoma (Figure 5.1) and related tumours. It also describes a spectrum of diseases, including hydatidiform mole, invasive mole, choriocarcinoma and placental-site tumour. Until 30 years ago, choriocarcinoma had a dismal prognosis. This has fortunately changed and it is now one of the most curable gynaecological malignancies. This is due to the fact that the tumour is chemosensitive, and has a sensitive and specific tumour marker, beta-human chorionic gonadotrophin (beta-HCG), allowing the identification of individuals at risk and the possibility of aggressive treatment with chemotherapy, surgery and radiotherapy.

Hydatidiform mole

The incidence of this condition varies geographically. In the UK and USA, it occurs in 1 in 1200 pregnancies. Its incidence is, however, much higher in the Far East, with reports suggesting it affects 1 in 77 pregnancies in some areas. Maternal age influences incidence, with lowest incidence in the 20–29 age range, and highest incidence in mothers under 15, or over 40. The incidence does not, however, appear to be related to parity, contraception or irradiation.

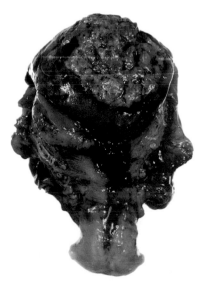

Hydatidiform mole can either be complete or partial. Complete mole carries an increased risk of progression to GTN compared with partial mole. Complete moles require chemotherapy in approximately 7% of patients, while only 3% of partial moles require chemotherapy. Partial moles account for approximately 10–15% of the total

Figure 5.1 Choriocarcinoma arising from uterine body.

incidence. In complete moles, no fetus is present and the placenta is composed entirely of vesicular tissue. In contrast, a fetus is present in partial moles, together with some normal placental tissue.

A normal karyotype is present in the complete mole – usually 46XX but occasionally 46XY. An empty egg is fertilized and the male haploid set reduplicates to create the diploid 46XX. Occasionally, two sperm, one carrying 23X and the other 23Y jointly fertilize the empty egg giving the diploid 46XY. In a partial mole, the fetus usually dies in the first or second trimester, and there is often a triploid karyotype.

Patients usually present with delayed menses, signs of pregnancy, perhaps vaginal bleeding or passage of vesicular tissue per vaginum. In addition, these patients are at greatly increased risk of developing pre-eclampsia and hyperthyroidism. Diagnosis is strongly suggested by ultrasound scanning and many moles are now picked up at routine antenatal scanning. The diagnosis of a hydatidiform partial mole may be made on ultrasound, but is often made only when aborted material is examined histologically. Measurement of beta-HCG will reveal an elevated level, but this can also occur in normal pregnancy.

Management. As described above, the diagnosis may be made either pre- or post-evacuation. When a diagnosis is made pre-evacuation, evacuation should be performed with suction curettage. For patients with a grossly enlarged uterus, laparotomy facilities should be available, although a hysterotomy or hysterectomy is only rarely required. Follow up after evacuation should follow the plan shown (Table 5.1).

GTN

GTN is preceded by a normal pregnancy in 25% of patients, and an abortion or ectopic pregnancy in 25%. Fifty per cent of GTN arises spontaneously following fertilization and is in the form of a hydatidiform mole. GTN has been classified according to the criteria shown in Table 5.2, and WHO scoring and FIGO staging systems exist.

Investigations for women with GTN include:

- full history
- examination
- chest X-ray

TABLE 5.1

Post-evacuation follow up for the management of hydatidiform moles

- Measurement of beta-HCG levels every 1–2 weeks until negative on two occasions, then bimonthly for 1 year. Contraception should be used for 6–12 months; the combined oral contraceptive pill is not contraindicated

- Physical examination including pelvic examination every 2 weeks until remission, then every 3 months for 1 year

- Chest film initially. Repeat only if the beta-HCG titre plateaus or rises

- Chemotherapy started immediately if:

  – the HCG titre rises or plateaus during follow up

  – metastases are detected at any time

Modified from DiSaia and Creasman, 1993

TABLE 5.2

GTN classification

Stage

I Non-metastatic disease: no evidence of disease outside the uterus

II Metastatic disease: any disease outside the uterus

    A. good prognosis metastatic disease

       1. short duration (last pregnancy < 4 months)

       2. low pretreatment HCG titre (< 100 000 IU/24 hours or < 40 000 mIU/ml)

       3. no metastasis to brain or liver

       4. no significant previous chemotherapy

    B. poor prognosis metastatic disease

       1. long duration (last pregnancy > 4 months)

       2. high pretreatment HCG titre (> 100 000 IU/24 hours or > 40 000 mIU/ml)

       3. brain or liver metastasis

       4. significant previous chemotherapy

       5. term pregnancy

Adapted from Hammond et al. 1973

TABLE 5.3

GTN recurrence

Disease	Remission (%)
Non-metastatic	100
Good prognosis metastatic	100
Poor prognosis	66
Total	92

Disease stage	Recurrence (%)
Non-metastatic	2.1
Good prognosis metastatic	5.4
Poor prognosis metastatic	21.0

Data from Hammond *et al.* 1980

- pretreatment beta-HCG
- full blood count
- urea
- electrolytes
- liver function tests

If any of these are abnormal, then a CT scan of the brain and ultrasound scans of the pelvis and liver should be performed. Treatment regimens are outside the scope of this book, but usually start with single-agent chemotherapy.

Prognosis. Recurrence of GTN is uncommon after chemotherapy (Table 5.3). Even when recurrence occurs, the results of further treatment are impressive. With modern chemotherapy, most patients with GTN can be cured, with most women retaining their uterus and fertility.

CHAPTER 6
Pain management and palliation

Prompt and effective management of pain is achievable for the majority of patients. For those with pain resistant to initial treatment, perseverance and referral to a specialist at a chronic pain centre is likely to result in improved quality of life.

Pain may be broadly divided into two distinct groups: nociceptive, which occurs where there is tissue damage, and neuropathic, which results from damage to, or an abnormality in the nervous system.

Cancer-associated pain

Cancer and pain are inextricably linked in the minds of patients and, unfortunately, many doctors. Pain in patients with cancer may be caused by the erosive effects of the tumour itself or by treatment (e.g. radiation plexopathy and constipation secondary to opioid drug administration). It may also result from muscle spasm or musculoskeletal problems arising from the consequences of the illness. The patient may, therefore, complain of various different types of pain.

Tumour erosion, muscle spasm and bony secondaries will produce nociceptive pain which may be sharp and stabbing, cramping or throbbing. Neuropathic pain produced by damage to the nervous tissue is characteristically shooting, lancinating, burning or described as feeling like electric shocks. It is often associated with paraesthesias and dysaesthesias.

Severity of pain may increase in proportion to either tumour mass or the occurrence of new metastases. A tumour enlarging within a fibrous capsule causes continuous pain which is gradual in onset, tending to start with an ache. Those involving a hollow viscus, such as the small intestine, interfere with peristaltic function and cause cramp-like or colicky abdominal pain. Tumours may become inflamed or infected, which will also produce pain; necrosis can occur subsequently, causing tenderness and pain.

Tumours can invade bone either by direct growth into it, or by distant metastases. Most gynaecological tumours do not usually metastasize to bone. In those that do, vulval and cervical carcinomas invade bone directly, and other tumours usually spread to this site by distant metastasis.

Nerve involvement. Tumours characteristically cause shooting or stabbing pain, radiating along the path of the nerve, both by direct infiltration but also by stretching or compressing nerves. The latter occurs particularly where the nerve lies against bone or within a bony cavity. For example, the lumbar and sacral plexuses may be infiltrated by primary and metastatic tumours in the pelvis, causing severe pain in the lower part of the back, pelvis and lower limbs. If the lower sacral plexus is involved, severe pain may be experienced in the perineum.

Isolated peripheral nerves, or their roots, may be affected by tumours in the pelvis. Involvement of the sciatic nerve, for instance, may produce pain radiating down the back of the leg into the foot. The lumbosacral plexuses may also be damaged by radiotherapy, producing radiation neuritis or plexopathy which may present with pain or sensory/motor deficits. Pain due to nerve involvement may be associated with sensory abnormalities such as dysaesthesiae or paraesthesiae. Patients may complain of, or present with motor or sensory deficits as well as pain.

Infiltration of the vascular system. Direct infiltration of arteries, veins and lymphatics occurs with gynaecological cancer, due to the close anatomical relationship in the pelvis. Arterial and venous involvement causes ischaemic pain and venous engorgement, respectively, distal to the blockage. Lymphatic involvement produces the distressing problem of lymphoedema distal to the blockage. Lymphoedema may be particularly painful and can easily be overlooked. Lymphoedematous legs are heavy to move and may cause pain by traction on intrapelvic structures.

Gastrointestinal symptoms. Hollow organs may be invaded by gynaecological tumours. If the bowel is involved, a cramping colicky pain may result. Bowel obstruction can be relieved by surgical resection of the involved segment; patients may require a colostomy and, if this is the case, will benefit from pre-operative counselling. Constipation and diarrhoea are also common problems for the patient with cancer.

Constipation often results from oral opioid therapy, so patients receiving opioid analgesics regularly should also be given laxatives. Faecal impaction is a potent cause of severe rectal pain. Good hydration and adequate levels of dietary fibre are, therefore, essential. For patients requiring laxatives, either bisacodyl 5–10 mg at night, or senna granules 5–10 ml at night, are useful. Failing this, glycerine suppositories and, for extreme cases, olive oil enemas and manual evacuation may be required.

Diarrhoea. Lomotil® (four tablets initially, then two tablets 6-hourly until relief occurs) or Imodium® (4 mg initially, then 2 mg after each loose bowel motion until relief occurs) are used at first. If this is not effective, codeine phosphate, 30 mg orally, three or four times a day, or by intramuscular injection (15, 30 or 60 mg), can be used.

Dry mouth/oropharynx. During cancer or its treatment, the patient's mouth and oropharynx can become dry, causing much discomfort. This can be relieved by mouthwashes, sucking on ice cubes or acid sweets, or by chewing gum. It is also important to counter dehydration and prevent infection. Maintaining good oral and dental hygiene can do much to prevent infection. Prompt treatment of oral candidiasis with nystatin lozenges or suspension can avoid a great deal of discomfort.

Hiccups are a gastrointestinal side-effect that can cause much distress; they may be relieved by inhaling carbon dioxide (i.e. by breathing into a paper bag). If this fails, chlorpromazine hydrochloride, 25 mg orally, three times daily, is usually effective. Alternatively, amphetamine sulphate, 2.5–5 mg three times daily, or hyoscine hydrobromide, at a starting dose of 300 mg which is repeated 2 hours later, can be used.

Nausea and vomiting may be caused directly by the tumour, by chemotherapy and radiotherapy or by opioid medication. Ondansetron is probably the drug of choice, 8 mg orally twice daily or 4 mg intravenously every 6 hours, otherwise metoclopramide can be used, 10 mg three times daily or administered intravenously with chemotherapy. Promethazine hydrochloride, 20 mg at night and 10 mg in the morning, can also be useful.

Urinary tract problems

Involvement of the urinary tract causes pain in the loin and groin that may range from a dull ache to colic. Cervical tumours often cause hydronephrosis and fistula formation. Ureteric blockage may be relieved by removal of the compressing tumour, or using ureteric stents. Nephrostomy tubes can be used if it is impossible to pass either antegrade or retrograde ureteric stents. These techniques are also useful for patients who require palliative urinary diversion as a result of cancer causing urinary fistulas. Occasionally tumours can cause urethral obstruction resulting in complete retention and this must be relieved by catheterization. Prompt recognition and treatment of urinary tract infection is also important in relief of associated pain, and in the prevention of ascending infection with its risk of pyelonephritis.

Radiotherapy

The dose of radiation used in radiotherapy is calculated to provide the maximum dose to the tumour while giving the least damage to the skin, contiguous tissues and organs. Radiation may cause tissue fibrosis involving the sacral and lumbar plexuses, causing sensory and motor deficits and neuropathic pain. The pain may be exacerbated by movements that stretch or produce tension in the nerve roots. Skin reactions occur during radiotherapy causing burning pain, which can be alleviated using 0.1% hydrocortisone cream or topical local anaesthetic creams.

Chemotherapy

Chemotherapy can cause pain both through direct cytotoxic activity and the production of peripheral neuropathy. For example, vincristine can cause tingling and numbness in the fingers and toes. The pain in peripheral neuropathies often decreases with time, but it may be quite disabling and refractory to treatment. Antidepressants may be of great benefit in this setting.

Both vincristine and vinblastine can cause myalgia and arthralgia, while procarbazine and 5-fluorouracil can cause neurotoxicity. All cytotoxics can cause mucosal reactions in the gastrointestinal tract – symptoms relate to the lips, mouth, pharynx, stomach and colon. Mucositis may be intensely painful and difficult to treat. Local anaesthetics, as lozenges, linctus or aerosols can be helpful in its treatment.

Lymphoedema

Lymphoedema is a troublesome condition in patients with cancer and occurs in 5–10% of women with vulval cancer. It also presents occasionally in patients after treatment of cervical and endometrial neoplasia.

Lymphoedema should be treated by elevation and the use of graduated compression bandages. Low-dose antibiotics should be used prophylactically in patients suffering from intermittent infection of oedematous legs.

For patients with more troublesome symptoms, intermittent positive pressure boots (Figure 6.1) can be used for 1–2 hours during the day to reduce the volume of lymph.

Pain relief

Curative cancer treatment – either by surgery, radiotherapy or chemotherapy – usually gives relief from pain that is being caused directly by the tumour. Even where such measures may not be curative, they may be invaluable in palliative pain management where pain is not easily controlled by standard measures. Indeed, radiotherapy will be the treatment of choice in certain circumstances such as isolated bone secondaries.

Effective postoperative analgesia is particularly important following oncological surgery as persisting pain is associated, in the minds of patients, with persisting cancer. Many centres now use epidural anaesthesia in the peri-operative period following major gynaecological surgery. Patient-controlled and continuous intravenous administration of opioid drugs have also improved the quality of postoperative analgesia.

The fundamental principles of analgesic therapy for patients with gynaecological (or any other) malignancy is that analgesics should be

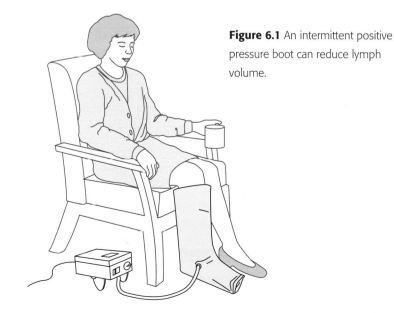

Figure 6.1 An intermittent positive pressure boot can reduce lymph volume.

prescribed for pain and the dose should be titrated to the patient's response. There is no merit in prescribing an inadequate dosage (as assessed on body weight) given infrequently with the aim of avoiding 'addiction'. There is no evidence that the administration of opioids in large enough doses to produce pain relief carries any appreciable risk of addiction.

Patients receiving strong painkillers will often need some time to determine the drug dose that adequately controls their pain. When this dose has been established, they may be controlled on a stable-dose regimen with regular review. Increasing dose requirements do not necessarily mean that tolerance to opioid drugs has developed. It may indicate progression of established disease or the development of new disease.

Pain in patients with malignancy may not be due to the underlying disease. Up to 30% of patients presenting with a diagnosis of cancer have been found to have pain unrelated to the underlying condition. The pain results from treatment in approximately 5% of cases, concurrent disorders such as osteoarthritis or migraine in 22%, and relates to debilities such as bedsores in 6% of patients. Pain diaries kept by patients and the use of visual analogue pain scores may help in the provision of effective analgesia.

Analgesic drugs may be divided into non-opioid, opioid and adjuvant or non-conventional analgesic drugs. Opioids are drugs that produce analgesia by binding to opioid receptors in the brain and spinal cord. The term 'opioid' should be used instead of the older, less descriptive, term 'narcotic'. It is unlikely that the patient with pain resulting from gynaecological malignancy (with or without metastatic disease) who has not had a curative operation, will be effectively treated without recourse to opioid analgesic drugs, alone or in combination. The use of opioid analgesic medication should not be seen as a last resort, nor should it be reserved until pain is intolerable. Early and effective analgesia improves the quality of patients' lives and may possibly improve longevity. WHO has produced a three-step analgesic ladder for cancer pain control (Figure 6.2).

Non-opioid analgesics include paracetamol, aspirin and non-steroidal anti-inflammatory drugs (NSAIDs). Paracetamol is a good minor analgesic that does not cause gastrointestinal problems but does not have an anti-inflammatory action. Aspirin has anti-inflammatory properties and may be helpful for treating non-visceral pain. Stronger analgesia with anti-

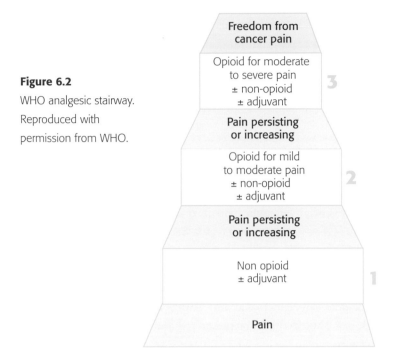

Figure 6.2

WHO analgesic stairway.
Reproduced with
permission from WHO.

inflammatory effects can be provided by NSAIDs such as indomethacin,
diclofenac and ketorolac. All the NSAIDs cause gastrointestinal irritation,
which may lead to gastric ulceration and haemorrhage. There is no
convincing evidence that the route of administration of NSAIDs alters the
incidence of gastrointestinal side-effects. They may reduce renal function
which, in some individuals, can lead to renal failure; this occurs more
commonly in the elderly. There may also be exacerbation of reversible airways
obstruction in susceptible individuals. Despite these side-effects, this class of
drug may be very effective, particularly in the treatment of bony metastases.

Tramadol hydrochloride is a synthetic opioid drug that inhibits
noradrenaline and serotonin uptake. It is used extensively in countries where
there are restrictions on opioid prescription and may be of value in the
treatment of cancer pain where patients are resistant to using morphine or
similar drugs.

*Opioids.*When non-opioid drugs fail to give a patient effective pain relief,
as is often the case with moderate and severe pain, opioid analgesia should
be started. Patients should be started on weaker agents but if these fail to

give satisfactory relief, attending physicians should have no hesitation in promptly switching to appropriate doses of stronger opioids.

For intermediate pain that has failed to respond to NSAIDs, codeine 30–60 mg every 4 hours, or dihydrocodeine 30 mg every 4–6 hours, can be used. These drugs, which all tend to cause constipation, should be taken after food.

If codeine or dihydrocodeine fail to relieve pain, morphine and, if available, diamorphine can be used. Morphine can be given in a slow-release tablet formulation (10, 30, 60 or 100 mg morphine sulphate tablets are available). If patients are in severe pain, the daily dose of morphine required may be determined by allowing the patient to self-medicate using oral morphine linctus taken hourly as required. It may also be delivered by patient-controlled intravenous infusion. The amount of morphine used over 24 hours can be calculated and an initial daily or twice-daily dose derived. Alternatively, when the patient is not in hospital, an estimated dose can be chosen and the dose can be increased until pain is relieved. Doses for breakthrough pain should always be prescribed and patients should never be unable to self-medicate in the event of an increase in pain. As already stated, an increase in analgesic requirement is more likely to result from progression of the disease than from any tolerance developing.

Antidepressant drugs are used widely in the management of chronic pain. They are the only drugs of proven value in the treatment of post-herpetic neuralgia and may well be useful in patients with neuropathic pain due to malignancy or its treatment (Table 6.1). The older tricyclics may be more effective in this role than the selective serotonin re-uptake inhibitors (SSRIs), such as fluoxetine or paroxetine. Exactly how antidepressants work in the treatment of pain is not fully understood. Modulation of descending cortical inhibitory pathways, positive effects on mood, and changes in central spinal processing have all been suggested as modes of action.

Anticonvulsant and membrane-stabilizing agents. Anticonvulsant drugs such as carbamazepine, and membrane-stabilizing agents such as lidocaine and mexiletine may be of benefit in alleviating neuropathic pain (Table 6.1).

Steroids. Intravenous steroids may be tried where pain is due to swelling of

TABLE 6.1

Adjuvant analgesic drugs in cancer pain relief

Class	Drug	Approximate daily dosage	Route
Tricyclic antidepressants	Amitriptyline hydrochloride	10–150 mg	PO/IM
	Clomipramine hydrochloride	10–150 mg	PO
	Desipramine hydrochloride	10–150 mg	PO
	Doxepin	12.5–150 mg	PO/IM
	Imipramine hydrochloride	12.5–150 mg	PO
SSRIs	Fluoxetine	20–60 mg	PO
	Paroxetine	10–40 mg	PO
Anticonvulsants	Carbamazepine	100–1200 mg	PO
	Clonazepam	2–10 mg	PO
Membrane stabilizers	Mexiletine	150–1000 mg	PO

the tumour. They may be of particular benefit for intracranial metastases and spinal cord compression. Intravenous dexamethasone, 4–10 mg, 4–6-hourly, appears to be the drug of choice.

Alternative therapies. Transcutaneous electrical nerve stimulation, acupuncture, aromatherapy, hypnotherapy and psychological therapies can all be helpful in the management of malignant pain.

Interventional pain management techniques. Where conservative management techniques have failed, patients should be considered for more invasive techniques of pain control. These might include nerve blocks, epidural/intrathecal administration of drugs and neurodestructive procedures. Such patients should be referred to a specialist pain management unit. An algorithm for the management of continuing pain in patients with cancer is shown in Figure 6.3.

Figure 6.3 Managing continual pain in patients with cancer.

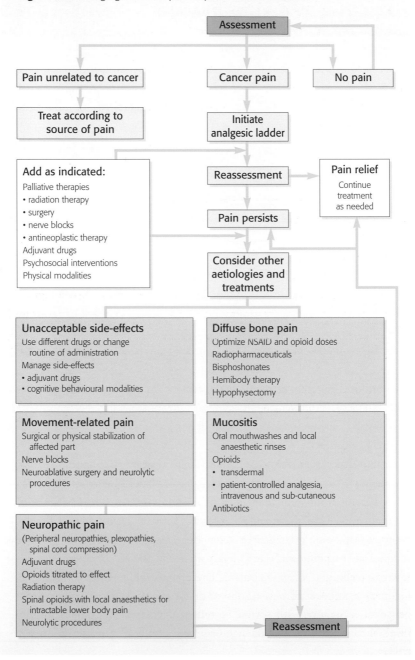

CHAPTER 7
Future trends

Developments are likely to occur in the areas of screening and chemotherapeutic regimens. There is an increasing trend towards management tailored to the individual, with the general aim of minimizing surgery while maximizing cure rate.

Cervical neoplasia

Current screening programmes are based on the original Papanicolaou methodology. However, great strides forward have been made in reducing laboratory errors. While not replacing the laboratory technicians, the recent introduction of computerized slide review systems has provided a useful means of double checking results.

In the USA, the availability of kits to type HPV has meant that HPV typing can be included with cytology. This may mean that gynaecologists will be able to predict more accurately which CIN lesions will progress and which are more likely to regress.

In the surgical arena, it seems likely that fertility-sparing procedures will become more widespread, particularly for women with small-volume tumours. For women with more advanced tumours, the combination of chemotherapy, radiotherapy and surgery may improve prognosis.

Ovarian neoplasia

The most exciting prospects are in screening. Women with a family history are already routinely screened; hopefully this will become available to all women in the not-too-distant future. While the recognition and increasing commercial availability of genetic testing is likely to create many ethical dilemmas in the short term, it is to be hoped that these will prove beneficial.

Chemotherapeutic regimens continue to improve, both in terms of efficacy and side-effects. The relatively recent addition of paclitaxel to regimens has proved useful. Paclitaxel in combination with cis-platinum is beneficial in women with advanced ovarian cancer, irrespective of surgical result. Carboplatin combined with paclitaxel may well prove to be equally efficacious.

Vulval neoplasia

Nowadays, vulval neoplasia appears to present more commonly in younger women than in previous times. This may be due to increasing levels of HPV and, possibly HSV infection. The epidemiological trend is likely to stimulate basic research into the aetiology of VIN progression. Surgical management is certainly moving towards more conservative surgery, and new methods of detecting lymph node involvement are being researched.

In conclusion

While much remains to be done in the field of gynaecological oncology, the explosion in research over the last 20–30 years has reaped rich dividends for our patients. This is reflected in increased survival times and increasing cure rate. In addition, prevention rates of both cervical and endometrial cancer are increasing as a result of treatment of ascertained precursor lesions. It is to be hoped that this trend continues.

Key references

GENERAL
Burghardt E, Tamussino K, Anderhuber F. *Surgical Gynecologic Oncology*. New York: Thieme Medical Publishers, 1993.

DiSaia PJ, Creasman WT. *Clinical Gynecologic Oncology*. St Louis: Mosby Year Book, 1993.

Gallup DG, Talledo OE. *Surgical Atlas of Gynecologic Oncology*. Philadelphia: WB Saunders, 1994.

Hammond CB, Weed JC Jr, Currie JL. The role of operation in the current therapy of gestational trophoblastic disease. *Am J Obstet Gynecol* 1980;136:844–58.

Pettersson F, ed. *Annual Report on the Results of Treatment in Gynaecological Cancer*, vol 20; Stockholm: International Federation of Gynaecology and Obstetrics, 1988.

Raven RW. *A Practical Guide to Rehabilitation Oncology*. New York: Parthenon Publishing, 1991.

Smith JR, Del Prioro G, Curtin J, Monaghan JM. *An Atlas of Gynaecological Oncology*. London: Martin Dunitz: In press.

CERVICAL AND VULVAL CANCER
Shepherd JH. Cervical and vulva cancer: changes in FIGO definitions of staging. *Br J Obstet and Gynaecol* 1996;103:405–6.

ENDOMETRIAL CANCER
Rose PG. Endometrial carcinoma. *New Engl J Med* 1996;335:640–9.

GESTATIONAL TROPHOBLASTIC NEOPLASIA
Hammond CB, Borchet LG, Tyrey L *et al*. Treatment of metastatic trophoblastic disease: good and poor prognosis. *Am J Obstet Gynecol* 1973;115:451–7.

PAIN MANAGEMENT AND PALLIATION
Parris WCV, ed. *Cancer Pain Management, Principles and Practice*. Boston: Butterworth-Heinemann, 1997.

Twycross RG, Lack SA. *Symptom Control in Far Advanced Cancer: Pain Relief*. London: Pitman, 1983.

Index

How to order

This *Fast Facts* book is one of a rapidly growing series of concise clinical handbooks.

Current *Fast Facts* titles:
- Benign Gynaecological Disease
- Benign Prostatic Hyperplasia (second edition)
- Breast Cancer
- Diabetes Mellitus
- Endometriosis
- Erectile Dysfunction (second edition)
- Gynaecological Oncology
- Hypertension
- Infection Highlights (published annually)
- Osteoporosis
- Prostate Cancer
- Prostate Specific Antigen
- Rheumatology Highlights (published annually)
- Schizophrenia
- Urinary Continence
- Urology Highlights (published annually)

For an up-to-date list of other titles
in this series or an order form,
simply phone or fax:

Phone: +44 (0)1235 523 233
Fax: +44 (0)1235 523 238